HOW TO LIVE A PERFECT LIFE :

Simple Tips to Live Happily and Healthy Without Medical Involvement.

Steven D. Guerrero

Table of content

Chapter 1

Eat nourishing food

We all understand that eating nutritious food is essential for good health, but it's usual to think of healthy eating primarily as a weight-loss strategy. However, the 2015 Dietary Guidelines for Americans state that for maximum energy, you should eat a balanced diet that is rich in fruits, vegetables, lean protein, low-fat dairy, and whole grains. After all, to some extent, you are what you consume. To acquire a variety of nutrients that will keep you energized throughout the day, eat from all the food categories. Choose fresh or frozen produce, especially the nutrient-dense dark leafy greens like broccoli and carrots, as well as orange veggies like sweet potatoes and carrots. Healthy protein options include a variety of fish and legume varieties. Eat 3 ounces of whole-grain pasta, bread, rice, or cereal each day.

The term "clean eating" recently became popular in the wellness community.

There is no clear definition for the phrase, and each person's interpretation varies. It has positive and uplifting implications for some people, while it has negative connotations for others, suggesting that the antithesis of clean eating must therefore be "dirty."

This viewpoint endorses the dichotomy between "good" and "bad" foods, or "healthy" and "unhealthy," which we don't believe is very useful when trying to develop a holistic and balanced perspective on health and food.

Undoubtedly, certain foods are better for your health than others. We couldn't say whether Mars Bars and broccoli have an equivalent impact on our health. But rather than what we do occasionally, it's more about what we do the majority of the time. Later on, we'll talk more about that.

BePure's guiding principle is essentially "just eat genuine food," which is the basis of "clean eating." Here is what we mean when we use those words so that everyone is clear:

The short answer is that, for us, a diet consisting of nutrient-dense, whole foods is what is meant by "clean eating."

Here is the lengthy response, beginning from the beginning, because it is only the tip of the iceberg:

The Pure Philippism

In line with our philosophy, you should eat nutrient-dense whole foods to promote your health while preventing sickness and inflammation.

Consuming a lot of fresh seasonal vegetables, fish, free-range eggs, nuts, seeds, organic grass-fed meat, soaked gluten-free whole grains, and legumes fall under this category.

It's more about plenty and less about constraints.

Foods like gluten, refined grains, some types of dairy, refined sugars, and highly processed vegetable oils don't fit our concept of "clean eating."

Because we don't think being dogmatic about this is helpful, we like to combine our clean eating philosophy with the "80/20 rule." A holistic sense of wellness requires flexibility.

Although we don't always steer clear of foods that are high in sugar, alcohol, or other undesirable ingredients, they make up 20% of our diet.

There is so much more to being healthy than just what you put in your mouth. As a result, being healthy may also mean celebrating a birthday with friends over cake and wine, as long as you don't make it a habit.

Although you will see that eating healthy food may be delectable and delightful, our goal is to provide you with the most energy, health, and vitality to enable you to live the life you want. This is what eating healthily 80% of the time promotes.

It can be beneficial to keep in mind the phrase "progress not perfection" while starting to incorporate more nutrient-dense foods into your diet.

More effective and long-lasting than trying to completely transform your lifestyle all at once are small, persistent modifications.

The advantages of consuming whole foods

1. Prevention of Inflammation

The ability of our body to control and regulate inflammation is supported by whole meals.

Trans-fats, refined grains, sugar, preservatives, and emulsifiers are food additives that can cause gastrointestinal dysfunction, memory loss, fuzzy thinking, chronic pain, and poor sleep.

Feeling drowsy and lethargic after eating pizza for lunch is probably something you have personally experienced.

What is inflammation, exactly?

The body employs inflammation to restore damaged tissue, heal itself after an injury, and fight itself against outside invaders like viruses and bacteria.

This is a normal and healthy reaction, but when our bodies experience persistently high levels of inflammation, it becomes difficult to feel joyful, healthy, and energetic. Over time, this can also result in pretty serious sickness.

2. Stabilizing Blood Sugars

Whole foods can keep blood sugar levels constant.

You typically feel more satisfied after eating because whole foods have a lower glycemic load—the rate at which your body converts the food into energy. In addition to being important for treating metabolic diseases including type 2 diabetes as well as weight management and modifying body composition, this can aid with cravings and energy.

Because each of our bodies is different, we need varied meal combinations to feel our best. To learn which foods support satiety and stable blood sugar levels the best, you can take the BePure Macronutrient Profile Questionnaire.

3. Increase Nutrient Uptake

When prepared properly, whole foods have a reduced level of anti-nutrients, which makes it easier for your body to absorb and utilize the nutrients from your diet.

When consumed, proteins from some foods may prevent the absorption of other nutrients. For instance, it has been demonstrated that when consumed with foods high in these nutrients, the proteins included in gluten-containing foods inhibit the absorption of iron, calcium, zinc, and magnesium.

This implies that if you habitually ingest gluten, even if you eat a healthy diet or take nutritional supplements, your body may not be able to keep or absorb these nutrients.

Inflammatory foods

As was already said, following a diet high in whole foods is good for your health.

Vegetables, soaking whole grains, legumes, meat, eggs, fish, nuts, and seeds are what we add, but they only make up a portion of the equation. Your health depends just as much on what we leave out.

Here are three typical foods that we advise avoiding as much as possible. Keep in mind that everybody is different.

Other things, including dairy and whole grains devoid of gluten, will fully depend on your specific tolerance. We advise starting with the three listed below because trying to modify everything at once can be overwhelming:

1. Gluten

For many people, grains, especially those containing gluten, can worsen conditions ranging from joint discomfort, weight gain, migraines, and thyroid problems to issues with digestion, mood, and skin conditions like rashes and eczema.

We have yet to see a thyroid patient at our BePure Clinic whose symptoms have not significantly improved on a gluten-free diet.

Check out this list for a comprehensive list of symptoms connected to gluten. You'll notice that a surprising number of these symptoms have nothing to do with digestion!

Starting a gluten-free diet can be perplexing at first. But once you get into it, you'll discover that there are still a ton of delicious, nutrient-dense, and less inflammatory alternatives.

Your body can be nourished without the inflammatory effects of gluten by eating foods like starchy vegetables, legumes, fruit, and soaked whole grains.

2. Refined Grains

Refined grains are heavily processed, stripped of their nutrients, and boost blood sugar levels.

Examples include pasta, wheat, morning cereals, crackers, processed bread, and biscuits.

Unexpectedly, cereals like corn flakes and rice bubbles have a higher glycemic index than regular table sugar!

Depending on your particular genetic makeup, a certain amount of carbohydrate is essential for both energy production and brain function. However, entire food sources including root vegetables, fruit, legumes, and soaking gluten-free grains provide all the advantages of complex carbs.

Concentrated consumption of refined grains can cause type 2 diabetes, insulin resistance, metabolic dysregulation, poor digestion, and weight gain.

3. Refined sugar

What we already knew—that we consume far too much sugar—has been proven by World Health Organization (WHO) research.

On average, New Zealanders consume 37 teaspoons of sugar every day!

That is approximately 34 teaspoons more than what BePure advises and 31 teaspoons more than the amount the WHO recommends.

When you eat sugar, your brain releases opioids, making you feel good and want more sugar. This is problematic since our livers were only intended to handle a little amount of the sugar molecule fructose.

In biological terms, humans have not advanced from earlier eras when fruit from the natural world served as our only source of sugar and served as an excellent source of nutrients and energy.

Nowadays, sugar is present in a wide variety of products, including pasta sauce, bread, cereals, canned vegetables, and even salt and vinegar chips (to counteract the vinegar!).

Our bodies are unable to keep up due to our exposure to processed foods, so the extra sugar is stored as fat in our bodies. Too much sugar can harm a variety of things, including your mood, blood sugar management, hormonal balance, fertility, and body composition.

Finding a healthy and satisfying eating style can take some time and experimenting, as we like to say. In the end, the diet that will keep you feeling satisfied for the longest emphasizes whole foods.

Chapter 2

Sleep Appropriately

Many people tend to need to work on developing the good habit of sleeping more. What keeps us from getting the minimum of seven hours of sleep each night that we already know we require? Consider how you might reduce the things that most disturb your sleep, and bear in mind that: Lack of sleep can exacerbate significant medical disorders and have a bad impact on your attitude, drive, and energy levels. One of the best things you can do to prepare yourself for a productive, energized day is to prioritize sleep.

A person needs a certain amount of sleep to maintain their health and wellbeing. Sleep is just as important to people's health as regular exercise and a balanced diet.

In the United States and many other nations, modern living does not often emphasize the importance of getting enough sleep. However, it's critical that people consistently attempt to get enough sleep.

The following are just a few of the many advantages that medical professionals believe getting a good night's sleep has.

1. Increased efficiency and focus

Getting enough sleep has been linked in studies to improved cognition, productivity, and focus.

In the early 2000s, researchers conducted several experiments to examine the consequences of sleep deprivation.

The researchers came to the following conclusions about the relationship between sleep and several brain processes:

A more recent study published in the Journal of Child Psychology and Psychiatry in 2015 found a direct correlation between children's sleep patterns and their conduct and academic achievement.

2. Lower risk of weight gain

Short sleep cycles and weight growth may be related, but the exact mechanism is unclear.

Numerous research over the years has found a connection between obesity and irregular sleep habits.

A more recent study, published in the journal Sleep MedicineTrusted Source, comes to the contrary conclusion that there is no connection between obesity and sleep deprivation.

This book contends that numerous earlier studies have inadequately accounted for additional characteristics, such as: consuming alcohol.

amount of physical activity, education, and type 2 diabetes lengthy working hours, long periods of inactivity.

A person's desire or capacity to maintain a healthy lifestyle may be impacted by sleep deprivation, but this may or may not directly contribute to weight gain.

3. Improved calorie control

There is evidence to show that getting a good night's sleep can aid a person in consuming fewer calories during the day, similar to how gaining weight does.

For instance, according to a study published in the Proceedings of the National Academy of Sciences of the United States of America (Reliable Source), sleep patterns alter the hormones that control appetite.

A person's body may be unable to properly manage their intake of food if they don't get enough sleep.

4. Greater athletic performance

A person's athletic performance can be improved by getting enough sleep.

The National Sleep Foundation states that individuals should get between 7 and 9 hours of sleep each night, while athletes may benefit from up to 10 hours. Therefore, getting enough rest is just as crucial for athletes as getting enough calories and nutrients.

The fact that the body heals while we sleep is one of the justifications for this requirement. Other advantages are:

- greater performance vigor
- increased vigor
- increased coordination and speed
- improved mental function

5. Heart disease risk is reduced

High blood pressure is a heart disease risk factor. The Centers for Disease Control and Prevention (CDC) Trusted Source states that obtaining enough sleep each night enables the body to regulate its blood pressure on its own.

By doing this, you can lower your risk of developing sleep-related illnesses like apnea and improve your heart health in general.

6. More emotional and social intelligence

Sleep and emotional and social intelligence are related. Lack of sleep makes it more probable for a person to struggle with reading others' facial expressions and emotions.

For instance, a study published in the Journal of Sleep ResearchTrusted Source examined how individuals react to emotional stimuli. The researchers came to the same conclusion as other earlier studies: little sleep reduces a person's capacity for emotional empathy.

7. Depression prevention

Research on the connection between sleep and mental health has been ongoing for a while. One conclusion is that sadness and sleep deprivation are related.

A study that will be published in JAMA PsychiatryTrusted Source looks at suicide death trends over a 10 years. It concludes that a lot of these deaths are caused by sleep deprivation.

According to another study published in the Australian and New Zealand Journal of PsychiatryReliable Sources, those who suffer from sleep disorders including insomnia are more prone to display depressive symptoms.

8. Lessen inflammatory

Getting enough sleep has been linked to a decrease in bodily inflammation.

For instance, a study published in the World Journal of GastroenterologyTrusted Source shows a connection between sleep deprivation and gastrointestinal disorders called inflammatory bowel illnesses.

The study showed that these illnesses can contribute to sleep deprivation, which in turn can contribute to these illnesses.

9. Increased immunity

The body can rejuvenate, heal, and restore itself while you sleep. This connection also applies to the immune system. According to certain research, the body can fight against infection with the aid of higher sleep quality.

However, more investigation into the precise mechanisms of sleep and how it affects the immune system of the body is still needed.

recommended times to sleep

More time spent outside can lead to better sleep.

Sleep needs vary from person to person, depending on their age. As a person ages, they typically require less sleep to function properly.

The breakdown, according to the CDC Trusted Source, is as follows:

0-3 months: 14-17 hours for newborns

4 to 12-month -old infants: 12 to 16 hours

Infant (birth to 2 years): 11–14 hours

3-5 years of age: 10-13 hours

6 to 12 years old: 9 to 12 hours

Teen (13 to 18): 8 to 10 hours

Adult (18 to 60 years old): 7+ hours

Adults (aged 61 to 64): 7-9 hours

Adults (age 65 and older): 7-8 hours

The type of sleep is just as significant as the quantity. Waking up in the middle of the night is a sign of inadequate sleep.

Even after getting a decent amount of sleep, you still don't feel rested.

A person can do the following to enhance the quality of their sleep:

Avoid sleeping in after getting ample rest.

a consistent time for bedtime each night.

being more active during the day and spending more time outside.

exercising, going to therapy, or using other methods to reduce stress.

Every person's general health and well-being depend on sleep, which is a crucial but frequently disregarded aspect of that. Sleep is essential for the body's ability to recover and prepare for another day.

Getting enough sleep may also reduce your risk of developing heart disease, gaining too much weight, and becoming sick longer.

Chapter 3

Keep Company with Good People

Spend as much time as possible with those who make you feel good. Your excitement and vigor will increase as you make connections with people who are upbeat and share your interests. On the other hand, socializing with people you don't connect with, who have pessimistic outlooks, moan frequently, or make poor decisions, will only deplete your energy reserves. Choose the company you keep carefully.

Your life is greatly impacted by other people. According to American businessman and motivational speaker Jim Rohn, "You are the average of the five people you spend the most time with." With this in mind, you should consider the people you spend time with in the same manner that you consider your diet and exercise routine.

Some are parasites. They drain you of your joy, your energy, and perhaps even part of your material assets. You could compare spending time with them to eating nachos on the couch.

So what characteristics make someone "excellent" to hang out with? And what advantages come from being surrounded by these people?

"Good Folks"

Good people don't have to be saints, or at least they shouldn't. They might volunteer their time during the winter holidays to feed hungry children in Africa, or they might just prod you to go to the gym more frequently. You're looking for pleasant, joyful folks who make your life better. They include:

relatives and friends

Coworkers

Friends that hang out at the same coffee shop

They are the people that will motivate you to succeed, encourage you to be a better person, give you the drive to change for the better, and support you when you do.

Good people frequently exhibit productivity at work. They set up routines that they follow, are organized, and don't readily become diverted from the objective. All of this also makes you more productive!

It's crucial to understand that "good" does not equate to "alike." The same substance in excess can stifle growth. You desire variety and constructive disagreements. Diverse viewpoints can aid in your desire to sponge up knowledge that you should have.

Write Down the Characteristics of the People You Spend the Most Time With After Thinking About Who You Spend the Most Time With.

Would you describe them as optimistic? Happy?

Now consider how they operate and impact you.

Do they inspire confidence in your ability to accomplish your objectives?

Do they back you up?

Do you find them attractive?

Do you feel elated and rejuvenated after being with them?

You most likely already have the nice people you require around you if you responded "yes" to these questions.

What Does "Good" Mean to You?

Karl Marx once said, "The only people worth keeping in your life are those who make you happy, who make you laugh, who assist you when you're in need, and who care. Everyone else is just passing through."

All people are unique. Some things that may make you happy but not me. The definition of assistance may vary from person to person. Finding the right people for you is the key.

So, how do you go about doing that?

Keep in mind that opposites attract. You need to exude confidence and good feelings. You must also be authentic. This will help you find the proper folks for you. You might also need to work on forgiving others. It's time to let go of the bitterness and sadness that resentment only produces.

You are surrounded by life when there are wonderful people around you. You'll experience less stress and more joy in ordinary activities. Decide to start spending more time with the excellent people in your life starting today.

Chapter 4

Avoid News Overdose

The news is a crucial tool for staying informed about what's going on around the globe. It may be instructive, enjoyable, or even inspiring. Unfortunately, there are far too many instances of pain in the news. These tales have the power to distort your perception of reality and make you concentrate on your darkest anxieties rather than the beauty all around you. Even while you can't completely avoid these stories, try to limit your exposure whenever you can, especially during trying times.

There is more to "keep up with" than simply the Kardashians, which may come as a shock. Reading the news is like keeping up with this wacky family, which not many people recognize. Everyone enjoys reading about drama and gossip but despises participating in it, so the news is the ideal source for your daily fix. You hear about all the drama that is taking place in the corporate world, the entertainment sector, sporting events, and the realm of elections in addition to getting the most recent information on what is occurring across the globe. It's the best of all worlds since you get your daily fix of rumors while also picking up a few new facts about your surroundings. Although it is still vital to follow the news, you may still keep up with the Kardashians.

1. The news keeps you informed and offers valuable educational information.

How does watching "Keeping Up with the Kardashians" help you? It keeps you informed on what is happening in their world. You learn how theatrical they can all be, sure, but how does this apply to you? You can have a deeper understanding of regional, governmental, and international issues by keeping up with the news. You can distinguish yourself from people who are confused about current events by doing this. Your professors and bosses will value that.

2. It benefits to make room in your mind for novel concepts and ideas.

You can gain a better grasp of what's occurring across the world by reading the news or watching it every day. You're surrounded by a variety of folks. It's crucial to educate oneself on other cultures and current events in other societies. By doing this, you can help those around you and yourself get rid of common cultural prejudices.

3. It is a wise practice to adopt.

Contrary to Scott Disick's habits, reading the news is a beneficial habit that won't land you in treatment. Keeping up with the news stimulates your mind in the same way that going to the gym every day improves your health. The news can be enjoyed while lounging on your couch with a hot cup of coffee or tea, or you can utilize it as an educational study break. You can set aside time for the news numerous times throughout the day.

4. You can come to your conclusions.

You must form your perspective rather than base it on those of your family, friends, and peers when discussing how they feel about various topics. Being aware of your surroundings helps you think more critically. Before casting your vote, it's crucial to understand how each candidate feels about several issues related to the election. You should establish your thoughts and choose the candidate that will benefit you the most and who best represents your values.

5. gives you more subjects to discuss.

It is crucial to be aware of current events, whether they pertain to local elections, the entertainment or sports industries, or global news. Imagine speaking with your potential employer during office hours or at a cocktail party; being up-to-date on current events enables you to come up with more interesting conversation starters. You can develop a more comprehensive perspective by hearing multiple points of view when discussing current events with others.

Chapter 5

Regular Exercise

Do you often feel drained by the middle of the day? Have you ever become exhausted performing routine tasks like grocery shopping or housework? Contrary to popular belief, meeting the Physical Activity Guidelines for Americans' recommendation of 150 minutes per week of exercise can increase, not decrease, your energy level. How? Exercise reduces stress and tension, builds muscle, and increases endurance, which makes your body more capable of performing other physical activities or tasks more effectively.

Health benefits of regular exercise

Any age can benefit from regular exercise with many health advantages. The best aspect is that training schedules and wellness plans may be modified to match all levels of health. Although many individuals are aware that exercise can lead to weight loss or greater fitness, there are many other advantages to regularly exercising in your daily routine. With daily workout routines, you may practically improve your life, enhancing everything from your energy to your sex drive.

Finding the strategy that works best for you is essential since sustained exercise efforts will yield the finest results. Even if you only work out for 10 minutes, find activities and routines that you enjoy performing. You will feel more invigorated and content with yourself after engaging in even brief bouts of exercise. Additionally, exercise lowers stress levels, and any quantity is preferable to a sedentary lifestyle.

Here are 7 health advantages of regular exercise to encourage you to incorporate it into your daily routine.

1. Your view on life will improve with regular exercise. While many of us have heard of the euphoria or "runner's high" that athletes experience as a result of endorphins, everyone can benefit from regular exercise's positive effects on mood. After a stressful day, an energizing gym regimen or brisk stroll will help you feel better and less stressed. Regular exercise routines can improve your weight reduction program or help you shape your muscles, both of which can increase your

confidence and self-esteem. And even better, at least one study discovered that exercise of any intensity reduced depressive symptoms. Daily physical activity appears to be essential for managing stress, which supports life balance, productivity, and general happiness.

2. Exercise regularly to increase your energy. Because exercising results in more energy throughout the day, many proponents of fitness make it a habit. Regular exercise enhances your ability to take in oxygen and boosts circulation throughout your entire body. Your cardiovascular system grows more effective with time, and regular exercise increases muscle

strength and endurance. This potent mixture works together to raise your wellness level, which naturally generates more energy and makes daily tasks and activities feel simpler.

3. Consistent exercise helps you sleep better at night. In fact, according to The Sleep Foundation, a nonprofit organization that compiles evidence-based sleep studies, regular exercise over 4 to 24 weeks improves the quality and length of sleep for those with insomnia. However, you do not need to experience insomnia to benefit from exercise because all types of exercise, from light to intense, have a good effect on sleep quality. Regular exercise

can help you fall asleep and sleep through the night in addition to its stress-relieving effects.

4. Strength training and other regular exercise regimens can help you maintain strong bones and muscles. Strength or weight training enhances muscle protein absorption, which reduces muscular degeneration and promotes muscle growth. But the advantages go further than that. Regular exercise also promotes bone density, which is crucial for injury prevention at any age and the prevention of osteoporosis later in life.

5. Consistent exercise can safeguard your brain and memory. These acts will supply your brain with more oxygen and nutrients from your blood, much as exercise encourages an increased flow of oxygen and blood to boost cardiovascular health. This may be the reason why regular exercise is associated with enhanced cognitive and memory functions. A region of the brain responsible for learning and memory, the hippocampus, has been found to grow in size when regular exercise routines are incorporated into a person's daily wellness regimen. Exercise also increases resistance to chronic disorders like dementia and Alzheimer's disease, which is great

news if you want to safeguard your brain against these and other age-related ailments.

6. Utilize aerobic exercise and strength training sessions to maximize fat loss and maintain a healthy weight. In addition to a balanced diet, frequent exercise boosts your efforts to lose weight and keep it off by speeding up your metabolism so you can burn more calories. Most people who make the switch to a better diet cut their caloric intake, which may slow down their metabolism. However, physical activity can help increase your metabolism and make up for the deficit, giving you greater benefits overall. Combining cardio and strength training will

enhance your efforts to lose fat and build muscle, leaving you leaner and more sculpted.

7. Regular exercise will stimulate your sex life. Numerous studies have demonstrated that exercise increases sex desire, but better fitness also promotes a fulfilling sexual life. Men who included 160 minutes of exercise each week for six months saw improvements in erectile dysfunction, according to a scientific assessment of ten studies. Another study of postmenopausal women found a correlation between regular exercise and improved sexual function and desire. You'll be happier in all aspects of your

life if you make fitness and exercise a daily habit.

Along with the aforementioned advantages, regular exercise can also give your skin a healthy glow, lower your risk of developing chronic illnesses, and generally make you feel better. If lack of motivation is a problem, have fun with online dancing workouts or friend-led walks. Try a workout app like Yes if you want to challenge yourself or feel competitive. Fit for thrilling races where you may earn medals and gear, or take on a fitness challenge and stay inspired as you track your progress. Enjoy the health advantages of regular exercise and discover the different methods to incorporate training routines into your life.

Chapter 6

Doing What is Meaningful Everyday

What do you have a strong feeling about? Do you possess a unique talent that you'd like to develop further or show off to others? Every day, indulge in something you enjoy, even if it's only preparing a nutritious dinner or listening to your favorite music. You'll be able to use and reserve your energy in ways that will bring out the best in you if you put effort into the things that are most important to you.

Easy ways to give your days more meaning

Here are 11 easy methods to make your day more meaningful, whether or not you're one of those hopelessly depressed drones out there.

Make a day plan. Although being spontaneous can be nice, there's no disputing that arranging and preparing your day will benefit you greatly. Your routine will become more purposeful throughout the day if you add some structure to it.

It's always a good idea to plan, even for mundane tasks like remembering to top off the cat litter and pick up the dry cleaning, as doing so provides you plenty of time to organize your schedule. Additionally, you increase your chances of setting aside free time for yourself.

Set aside some cash. You'll be shocked by how much, over time, a dollar here and a fiver there may mean to you. Set away some cash in a piggy bank each day. Choose the kind that prevents you from accessing your money until you break it. That will prevent you from using money from your fund.

In a year, you'll be shocked to see how much money you have when you bust it open. Knowing that you have meaningfully saved some money for the near future will do you the world of good.

Try to be good. One of the best ways to give your day significance is to pay it forward. Don't call it a day until you've helped someone else. Giving your secretary the day off or purchasing a coffee for the person in line behind you are just a couple of examples. Another simple example would be giving up your seat on the metro.

Whatever you do, make sure it's for someone else. You'll be rewarded tenfold and in ways you never thought imaginable.

"I love you," you say. It will mean a lot to you and the person you are sending love and good thoughts to if you send them to someone you care about. At least once every day, tell your partner, children, parents, or best friend, "I love you." This will serve as a reminder that you have individuals in your life who care about you and, more importantly, that they are aware of your concern for them.

Try something terrifying. A while back, there was a social media fad pushing people to do something terrifying every day for an entire year. It might appear difficult, but it's not at all.

It doesn't imply that you must engage in risky pursuits like bungee jumping from a bridge or paragliding off of buildings. Even the simple things matter, like ordering a different beverage than your typical latte. Give your life some significant thrills by trying something new every day, whether it's quitting your job or asking an attractive graphic designer to work out.

Make an effort to smile. Making an effort to be joyful is another approach to give your day more significance. When you start to sense negative thoughts creeping in, push them away and think of joyful ones in their place.

The solution should be something straightforward, like laughing at a joke or looking at vacation photos. Your day will feel more significant if you choose to be positive for longer and more frequently.

Make somebody laugh. By trying to make someone smile, you can enrich your day in a similar way to paying it forward. You never know how much a small act of kindness can mean to someone, whether it's telling a stupid joke to your coworker at the water cooler or helping your neighbor with her groceries.

Do some yoga. You need to do yoga every day, as cliche as that may sound. I'm not suggesting you spend 90 minutes practicing Bikram hot yoga in its entirety. I'm talking about getting ready in the morning to some soothing music and performing three sun salutations.

Stretching won't necessarily give your day significance; instead, deep breathing and mind-stilling exercises before facing the day will.

Play this great song. I wholeheartedly concur with the notion that music nourishes the spirit. Make sure you listen to at least one fantastic song every day. Do that regardless of whether it's your favorite song or something new you discovered on Spotify or 8tracks.

If you can, join in the dancing! The song will not only brighten your day but also put you in a pleasant mood, which will let you realize how lovely and deserving of appreciation every day is.

Remind yourself how happy you are to be alive. It's amazing how many people require a reminder of this basic reality. You're able to wake up, leave your bed, and go about your day is a miracle. Millions, if not billions, of people worldwide, would give anything to be in your position.

Just keep telling yourself that life is lovely and that you are oh-so-lucky to be here, whether you're thinking about people who have terminal illnesses or those who live in areas of the world without any of the daily comforts you take for granted. The more you say it, the more likely it is that you'll realize, to your astonishment, that it is the truth in every aspect.

Think about why. Reminding yourself of your motivations for doing what you do is one of the best things you can do to make your day more meaningful. We all have reasons for doing what we do, no matter how much we hate it, whether it's saving money for that backpacking trip across South America or working hard to pay for your kids' college education.

Ask yourself, "Why are you doing this?" You can put up with everything that occurs to you once you understand why. There is no reason why you can't leave society's bandwagon, pack your bags, go on an adventure, and start doing something that will make you happy if you don't have a valid excuse.

You give yourself the chance to recognize and comprehend just how great life truly is by adding a bit more significance to your day. It's ultimately up to you to make each day count. Even though you are surrounded by joyful people, if you won't change your negative outlook on life, life won't necessarily follow suit. You'll start to feel much better if you begin to give your everyday routine some significance.

Chapter 7

Have Good Thoughts for Others

Another approach to saving energy is to keep a sympathetic attitude. Kind attention is a manifestation of this way of thinking. For instance, attempt to smile and make eye contact with a stranger while also wishing them well. Instead, this kind of deed might stop you from passing judgment on that individual. Judging others can lead to us judging ourselves as well, and that kind of critical internal debate can be draining.

The last thing you want to hear when you're feeling sad is the metaphor of the glass being half full. What does that accomplish for you?

There may not seem to be any advantage to thinking positively at that time. You were hoping for the full glass, therefore you're disappointed. Furthermore, you lack it. Or perhaps you feel as though your glass doesn't even exist. It's someone else's, broken, stolen, and shattered.

Spend some time with your negative emotions, such as anger, frustration, disappointment, sadness, and fear. It's important to acknowledge them before moving forward.

Life can be challenging and confusing. It can come across as very tone-deaf when someone urges you to "cheer up" or "think positively." Positive thinking without regard for reality is rarely helpful. Because of this, positive thinking has a bad reputation due to poisonous optimism.

Positive thinking that accepts reality may not produce any instant miracles, but it can ultimately be beneficial to all of us in the long run. Growth and hope are beneficial to your health.

Although some people are naturally more optimistic than others, it is still possible to develop an optimistic outlook on life.

What is positive thinking?

The first thing to understand about positive thinking is that it doesn't imply ignoring logic or facts or coercing yourself to feel just good feelings. That is not practical.

When you think positively, you maintain a positive attitude in the face of stressful circumstances or bad news. Instead of letting the crisis or setback consume you, you're able to look past it.

Even though you may need to confront and deal with the drawbacks, you know you will overcome them. You are aware that just because there is terrible news doesn't mean everything is awful or that nice thing will never happen to you again.

Instead of expecting the worst and leaping to negative conclusions, someone who thinks positively assumes that others have the best of intentions and interprets others' behaviors more positively. Optimistic thinkers can envision positive outcomes.

Self-talk is frequently the first step in positive thinking. We are always having thoughts in our heads. Some opinions may be based on unambiguous facts, but many also have a positive or negative outlook.

You're probably more pessimistic if you engage in more negative self-talk and dwell on all the drawbacks. But that doesn't mean we can't alter our actions to have a more optimistic outlook.

It takes some work, but if you practice deliberately thinking more positively, your brain will start to develop new thought patterns. Some optimists put a lot of effort into controlling their negative feelings, yet mindfulness and self-compassion can modify harmful thought patterns.

Advantages of optimistic thinking

Why is having a positive outlook important?

Your physical and mental health can be impacted by the power of positive thought. You might be surprised by the advantages of positive thinking for your health.

Read through this list of 10 advantages of positive thinking for your health and consider how they might affect your life:

- more effective stress management and coping mechanisms.
- reduced chance of depression
- more able to withstand the typical cold.
- reduced danger of heart attacks and cardiovascular disorders.
- decrease in blood pressure

- better at resolving issues.
- increased capacity for change.
- more original thought
- attitude that is constant and less moody.
- improved leadership abilities.

Positive thinking has many advantages, but sometimes it might be difficult to get started. Your BetterUp coach will assist in directing you toward developing more constructive self-talk. With BetterUp, you may begin to feel what it's like to have a coach who is committed to your development.

Five suggestions for "thinking positively"

It takes practice to maintain an optimistic outlook. If you have trouble thinking positively, realize that it will take time to entirely alter your self-talk habits. People who tend to think more negatively may find it difficult to alter their cognitive patterns.

It's critical to realize that it's normal to occasionally relapse into negative mental patterns. What counts is that you're making an effort to empower yourself to think more positively by becoming aware of your automatic negative ideas and rephrasing them in a more positive way.

Being conscious allows you to challenge your pessimistic automatic thinking. Many coaches advise using some variation of these inquiries to gauge your thinking:

Is it real? Is the sky falling or may there be another explanation?

Is it beneficial? Does this interpretation motivate me to come up with fresh ideas or assist me in navigating this situation effectively?

Is it decent? Does this way of thinking give me the confidence to ask for assistance or support from others?

Here are five other suggestions to get you thinking positively:

1. Always be appreciative

Being close to your family or the rain holding off while you walk to work are just two examples of the numerous major and small things in your life for which you might be thankful. Whatever you have to be thankful for, list it and put it in a gratitude diary. Think about the blessings in your life when you're feeling down or sad to lift your spirits.

2. Obtain adequate rest

Are you attempting to get enough sleep every night, if not already doing so? A good night's sleep prepares you for a successful day. It enables us to refuel and complete our tasks. It won't improve your mindset to dwell on your fatigue. So try creating a decent overnight routine that puts your sleep schedule first. Otherwise, your self-talk will be full of impatient ideas and a desire to get your day over with.

3. Take things as they are.

It makes no sense to act as though nothing happened while you're dealing with a bad circumstance. Reframe the issue, saying something like, "This provides me with the chance to get some exercise and fresh air," if, for instance, your brother has taken the car and you have to walk to an appointment.

Recognize your sphere of influence. Accept the things you can't alter and try to focus on the good things instead.

4. List the things you need to improve.

Is there a particular circumstance or setting that causes you to become excessively pessimistic? You can start developing tactics that will help if you can pinpoint the problems that interfere with your optimistic attitude toward life. Your commute to work can be the cause of your unfavorable thoughts.

Make an effort to enjoy the task. Next time, put together a lively music playlist to listen to on the way to work. Spend less time with those who sap your energy and more time with those who make you feel good.

5. Don't forget to laugh

It helps you see the positive side of things when you make an effort to find humor in everyday situations. You can also lower your heart rate and manage stress thanks to it. If you're unable to laugh, try smiling. You can accept any errors and relax by laughing together with yourself. If necessary, find a hilarious video to watch or contact a funny buddy.

www.ingramcontent.com/pod-product-compliance
Lightning Source LLC
LaVergne TN
LVHW050330160826
845677LV00014B/3571

* 9 7 9 8 8 4 7 3 7 8 5 8 1 *